365
WAYS
to Get Out the
FAT

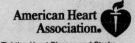

American Heart
Association.

Fighting Heart Disease and Stroke

365 WAYS

American Heart
Association®
Fighting Heart Disease and Stroke

to Get Out the

FAT

A Tip a Day
to Trim the
Fat Away

Clarkson Potter/Publishers
New York

Your contribution to the American Heart Association supports research that helps make publications like this possible. For more information, call 1-800-AHA-USA1 (1-800-242-8721) or contact us online at http://www.americanheart.org.

Published by Clarkson Potter/Publisher, New York, New York. Member of the Crown Publishing Group.

Random House, Inc., New York, Toronto, London, Sydney, Auckland
www.randomhouse.com

CLARKSON N. POTTER is a trademark and POTTER and colophon are registered trademarks of Random House, Inc.

Originally published by Times Books in 1997.

Printed in the United States of America

Art direction by Naomi Oshoe
Book design by Leon Bolognese & Associates, Inc.
Illustrations by David Cain

Library of Congress Cataloging-In-Publication Data
365 ways to get out the fat: a tip a day to trim the fat away.
American Heart Association.—1st ed.
    1. Low-fat diet.   2. Heart—Diseases—Diet therapy.
    I. American Heart Association
RM237.7.A176   1997
613.2'84—dc21   97-28430

ISBN 0-8129-6385-7

10 9 8 7

No book, including this one, can ever replace the advice of a physician. It's a good idea to check with your doctor before starting this or any other health program. Although we cannot guarantee any results, we hope this book will help you both attain your goals for better health and work more effectively with your doctor.

Preface

We know how it is: You want to eat less fat. You want to have a healthy heart. You want to reach or maintain a healthy weight. But you're *busy.* You don't have time to read a book the size of the Manhattan telephone directory to find out how to lower your cholesterol level.

Welcome to heaven. At the American Heart Association, in sympathy for your plight, we developed *365 Ways to Get Out the Fat,* a lightning-fast guide to slashing saturated fat and cholesterol from your diet. Sit back and fasten your seat belt. In 365 telegraphic tips, we give you everything you need to know to eat less fat—and help your heart last a lifetime.

Acknowledgments

They said it couldn't be done, but we did it!

At the American Heart Association, we know a lot about how to cut the fat in your diet. But did we know *365 ways*? Turns out we did. But it took a team effort to pull it off.

Managing Editor Jane Anneken Ruehl got the ball rolling by researching American Heart Association publications and other sources for ideas. Then she pulled together our team of experts, writers, and editors. Finally, she managed the development process from concept to completed book.

Writer Pat Naegele culled through tons of research to come up with the very *best* 365 tips we could possibly offer. She added verve and zip to each tip for a fun, readable book. Next, Editor Ann Melugin Williams took the completed manuscript and painstakingly copyedited every word. She checked the facts and polished it to perfection.

Meanwhile, Intellectual Properties Director Debra Ebel negotiated with the publisher and skillfully handled many of the business aspects of getting this book into your hands. And Editorial Assistant Marquel Huebotter stayed in high gear, inputting corrections, corralling camera-ready art, and handling the dozens of details necessary to get a finished manuscript to the publisher.

But all of our efforts would have been for nothing without Senior Science Consultant Mary Winston, Ed.D., R.D., who carefully assessed each tip for scientific accuracy and nutritional savvy.

We hope that our work will give you a fast, easy way to reduce the amount of fat you eat every day. We know that following these tips can help change your health—and your future—for the better.

Contents

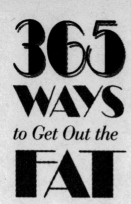

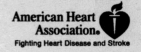

American Heart
Association.
Fighting Heart Disease and Stroke

365
WAYS
to Get Out the
FAT

Introduction

Secrets of the Food Pyramid

It doesn't take an archaeologist to see that Egyptians were on to something when they built the pyramid. It's a super-solid structure with a huge foundation and smaller and smaller rooms built above it.

The American Heart Association has borrowed this concept to create its Healthy Heart Food Pyramid. At a glance, it shows you the kinds and amounts of food to eat every day. It's easy to see that most of the pyramid is made up of two food groups: "Breads, Cereals, Pasta, and Starchy Vegetables" and "Vegetables and Fruits." Your diet should be the same—mostly made up of these foods. That's because they're naturally low in fat and high in nutrition. They're the foundation of your low-fat eating plan.

Exploring the next level, you'll see the "Skim Milk and Low-Fat Dairy Products" and "Lean Meat, Poultry, and Seafood" groups. These foods contain protein, calcium, and other nutrients, but you'll want to plan fewer servings of them because most of them contain quite a bit of fat.

Skim milk is an exception. The trend is to label skim milk "fat free" or "nonfat." So just remember that skim by any other name is still good for you.

Reaching the top of the pyramid, you'll find foods

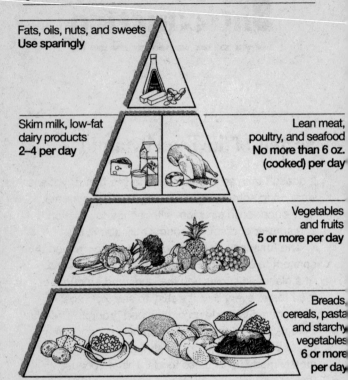

Fats, oils, nuts, and sweets
Use sparingly

Skim milk, low-fat
dairy products
2–4 per day

Lean meat,
poultry, and seafood
**No more than 6 oz.
(cooked) per day**

Vegetables
and fruits
5 or more per day

Breads,
cereals, pasta
and starchy
vegetables
**6 or more
per day**

we call "Now and Then"—foods you should have only
occasionally. These are fats, oils, nuts, and sweets.
They contain mostly fat and calories and few other
nutrients. The tip of the pyramid carries a curse: If
you eat too much of these foods, your waistline
expands and your cholesterol level could go through
the roof. So take a tip from us—go easy on these
foods.

The secret of the AHA Healthy Heart Food

Pyramid is simple. It's a tool to help you decide what kind of foods to eat and how much to eat every day. And that's a major discovery.

You Are What You Eat

The Law of Averages

You're at your favorite Northern Italian restaurant—foods taste just like they do in the old country. With a flourish, your waiter brings you Fettucine Pescatore in a bowl the size of a small dog. This is 1 serving of pasta, right?

Wrong. It's about 4. It may *seem* like a normal serving because that's what restaurants typically serve their patrons. But in truth, an average serving of pasta is about 1 cup. So you can see how easy it is to overeat without even knowing it.

To eat your healthiest, you need to know what an average serving is in each food group. That way, you won't be fooled into thinking that a jumbo bagel is only 1 serving. You'll know it's really 2 or 3 servings, and you can plan accordingly.

Breads, Cereals, Pasta, and Starchy Vegetables

This group is the greatest thing since sliced bread! It *is* sliced bread—and more. Adults and teens need 6 or more servings of this group per day. Preschool children and preteens need 4 servings. An average serving size is:

◆ 1 slice of bread

◆ 1/3 to 1/2 of a bagel

◆ 1 cup cooked rice or pasta

◆ 1 cup flaked cereal

◆ 1/4 cup nugget-type cereal

◆ 1/2 cup cooked cereal

◆ 1/4 to 1/2 cup starchy vegetables, such as potatoes or yams

Vegetables and Fruits

True statement: You need at least 5 servings of fruits and vegetables each day to help get the vitamins, minerals, and fiber your body requires. Yet, if you're like most Americans, you eat only 3 1/2 servings per day. Don't go bananas. Getting 5 servings of fruits and vegetables is not that difficult. Take a look at these serving sizes:

◆ 1 medium piece of fruit

◆ 1/2 to 1 cup cooked or raw vegetables or fruit

◆ 1/2 cup fruit or vegetable juice

Skim Milk and Low-Fat Dairy Products

Got milk? Good. Then follow the AHA's recommendation to have 2 to 4 servings of skim milk or nonfat or low-fat dairy products every day. For most people, 2 servings will do nicely. But for teens, pregnant or breast-feeding women, and everyone over age sixty-five, you need at least 3 servings a day. Note that children under age two should have whole milk. A serving size is

◆ 1 cup skim (fat-free or nonfat) or 1% fat milk

◆ 1 cup nonfat or low-fat yogurt

◆ 1 ounce nonfat or low-fat cheese

◆ 1/2 cup nonfat or low-fat soft cheese (e.g., cottage cheese)

Lean Meat, Poultry, Seafood, and Eggs

If you tend to pig out on meat, poultry, and seafood, you're not alone. The fact is, most people eat far too much protein. And along with that protein, they often get a hefty amount of fat. So don't be chicken about limiting the amount of protein you eat every day. It pays to keep these serving sizes healthy. A serving is

◆ 4 ounces raw lean meat (3 ounces cooked)

◆ 4 ounces raw poultry (3 ounces cooked)

◆ 4 ounces raw seafood (3 ounces cooked)

◆ 1 egg yolk (and no more than 3 or 4 egg yolks per week)

Now and Then Foods
(Fats, Oils, Nuts, and Sweets)

Is your sweet tooth taking a bite out of your low-fat game plan? It's easy to overeat when it comes to fats and sweets. How often do you use a 1/4 cup of salad dressing rather than just a tablespoon? Overdo it on the homemade chocolate chip cookies? Slather bread and potatoes with margarine? It's all easy, but it's not a good idea for your cholesterol level. Keep the tip-of-the-pyramid foods to a minimum in your diet—no more than 5 to 8 servings a day. Serving sizes for these foods are

◆ 1 teaspoon vegetable oil or margarine with no more than 2 grams of saturated fat per tablespoon

◆ 2 teaspoons diet margarine

◆ 1 tablespoon chopped nuts

◆ 1 tablespoon seeds without shells

◆ 1 tablespoon salad dressing

◆ 2 teaspoons mayonnaise

◆ 2 teaspoons peanut butter

◆ 10 small or 5 large olives

◆ 1/8 medium avocado

◆ 1 1/2 tablespoons sugar, syrup, jam, honey, or preserves

◆ 6 fluid ounces lemonade or sweetened carbonated beverage

◆ 3/4 ounce candy made primarily with sugar (e.g., gumdrops, mints, and hard candy)

◆ 1 slice angel food cake (1/24 of cake)

◆ 2 gingersnaps

◆ 1/3 cup fruit ice or sherbet

◆ 1/2 cup fruit-flavored gelatin

◆ 1 fig bar cookie

The ABCs of a Healthy Heart

Today's lesson: It's not enough just to cut the fat from your diet. In a way, that's easy. The tough part is to get all the nutrients your body needs for good health *while* you're eating less fat.

For example, you could eat only bread and fruit. Your fat intake would drop to almost nothing. But eventually, you'd become ill from lack of vitamins, minerals, and other nutrients. Balance is the key. Your homework? Eat a wide variety of nonfat and low-fat foods. This book will show you how.

Pop Quiz: What Is a Balanced Diet?

The answer is elementary. A balanced diet includes a variety of nutritious foods. We developed the following chart to show you a typical balanced diet. Take a look at how your current diet compares. Do you get enough of every food group? Do you eat 4 servings of meat every day but only 2 of vegetables?

Do You Eat a Balanced Diet?

Food Category	Recommended Number of Servings	The Number of Servings I Usually Eat Each Day (choose only one):		
		Too few	Right on	Too many
Breads, Cereals, Pasta, and Starchy Vegetables	6 or more per day	❑	❑	❑
Vegetables and Fruits	5 or more per day	❑	❑	❑

Food Category	Recommended Number of Servings	The Number of Servings I Usually Eat Each Day (choose only one):		
		Too few	Right on	Too many
Skim Milk and Low-Fat Dairy Products	2 to 4 for adults over 24 and children aged 2 to 10; 3 to 4 for ages 11 to 24 and women who are pregnant or breast-feeding	❑	❑	❑
Lean Meat, Poultry, Seafood, and Eggs	2 (no more than a total of 6 oz. of cooked lean meat, poultry, or seafood per day)	❑	❑	❑
	No more than 3 or 4 egg yolks per week	❑	❑	❑
Now and Then (Fat, Oils, Nuts, and Sweets)	Use sparingly		❑	❑

Final Exam: Learning to Take It One Tip at a Time

In this book, you'll find 365 tips for eating less fat. But don't attempt them all at once. That's like trying to get your MBA the first week you're at Harvard. Instead, start with the ones you find easiest. If you're a whole-milk fanatic, switch to 2%. After a couple of weeks, try 1% or skim. If you love eggs for breakfast, use 1 whole egg and 2 egg whites in your next omelet. One small step at a time. Easy does it.

As you begin substituting margarine for butter and bagels for croissants, you'll see how easy it is to pick up the habit of low-fat eating. And as these changes become habits, then you can add more. You'll also find that fat is a matter of taste. People who have gradually switched from high-fat to low-fat eating often say they now prefer the lighter, fresher taste of low-fat dishes. So taste is a matter of taste.

How to Graduate With Honors

Numero uno is to get support from your family. The AHA diet was originally developed for all healthy Americans over age two. That means almost anyone would benefit from it. So have your family and friends join you. And if they're not ready to join you, at least get their support.

Next, think positive. These tips don't tell you what *not* to eat. They tell you how to put together mouth-watering foods that are low in fat. They tell you how to substitute low-fat ingredients for high-fat ones while keeping the flavor and gusto. The AHA eating plan is a *good* thing. You'll never regret your decision to change your life—and possibly your health—by using these tips.

Then set yourself some goals. For every 10 tips you add to your life, reward yourself. Go to a movie, buy a CD, allow yourself time to read a new novel, or take a weekend trip. Be creative with these rewards. You deserve them.

Finally, realize that you will slip up. You'll go face down into Aunt Martha's homemade cheesecake. It's gonna happen. Your response? Immediately get back to your game plan. Because it's what you eat every day, not the occasional splurge, that determines your fat intake, your overall cholesterol level, and your heart's health. Simply get yourself back on track as soon as possible.

Reading Between the Lines: How to Find the Fat Content in Packaged Foods

Thanks to the nutrition labels now required on prepared foods, it's easy to figure out how much fat you're getting in a single serving.

Also there are many nonfat and low-fat versions of traditional foods available in your supermarket. You can use these to lower the fat content of your old family recipes and "comfort foods" to fit your new eating plan. But you need to read the labels for calories per serving. Don't think you can eat the whole box of nonfat brownies just because one brownie has less than 1 gram of fat! Your body has a way of turning excess calories into fat—just not as efficiently as fat into fat.

The sample nutrition label on page 13 clearly shows the serving size, number of calories, calories from fat, and the amount of total fat, saturated fat, and cholesterol in a single serving.

Nutrition Facts

Serving Size 1/2 cup (114g)
Servings Per Container 4

Amount Per Serving

Calories 90   Calories from Fat 30

% Daily Value*

Total Fat 3g	**5%**
Saturated Fat 0g	**0%**
Cholesterol 0mg	**0%**
Sodium 300g	**13%**
Total Carbohydrate 13g	**4%**
Dietary Fiber 3g	**12%**
Sugars 3g	
Protein 3g	

Vitamin A	80%	• Vitamin C	60%
Calcium	4%	• Iron	4%

*Percent Daily Values are based on a 2,000 calorie diet. Your daily values may be higher or lower depending on your calorie needs:

	Calories	2,000	2,500
Total Fat	Less than	65g	80g
Sat Fat	Less than	20g	25g
Cholesterol	Less than	300mg	300mg
Sodium	Less than	2,400mg	2,400mg
Total Carbohydrate		300g	375g
Fiber		25g	30g

Calories per gram:
Fat 9   •   Carbohydrate 4   •   Protein 4

Of course, if you eat double the amount of the serving size listed, you'll have to double the amounts of calories and fats, too.

High Hopes for Low Cholesterol

Dozens of scientific studies have shown conclusively that people with high blood cholesterol can switch to eating low-fat, low-cholesterol foods and reduce their blood cholesterol level.

What Is Fat?

Before you can fight fat, you have to know what it is. Basically, there are three types of fat in foods: saturated, polyunsaturated, and monounsaturated.

Saturated Fat

This is public enemy number one. Eating a lot of saturated fat usually sends your blood cholesterol level skyrocketing. Saturated fat is found mainly in foods of animal origin, such as meats, poultry, lard, butter, and whole-milk dairy products. It is also found in coconuts, palm, palm kernel oil, and cocoa butter. (These fats are often hidden in commercially baked goods, so be on the lookout.) Read labels and substitute similar foods that contain unsaturated fat.

Polyunsaturated Fat

This is one of the good guys. Polyunsaturated fats may help lower your blood cholesterol level when your diet is low in saturated fat. You'll find polyunsaturated fat in walnuts, corn oil, safflower oil, and fish.

Monounsaturated Fat

This is the superstar of fats. Widely used in both the Mediterranean and Japan (where heart disease is rare), this type of fat also may help reduce blood cholesterol in a low-saturated-fat diet. Foods that are high in monounsaturated fat are olive oil, canola oil, peanut oil, and avocados. But remember: Even when we talk about "good fat," we're not suggesting you add more fat to your diet. Your goal is to eat less fat overall and substitute monounsaturated and polyunsaturated fats for saturated fats whenever possible.

What Is Cholesterol?

Cholesterol is a waxy, fatlike substance that the body needs to make cell membranes and hormones. Dietary cholesterol is found only in foods of animal origin, such as egg yolks, meats, fish, poultry, and dairy products. In addition to the cholesterol you may get from food, your body also produces cholesterol. The amount you produce depends on the amount and kinds of fat you eat as well as on your genes.

If the combination of the cholesterol you eat and the cholesterol produced in your body overloads your system, it will accumulate on the inner walls of your arteries and clog them, which can lead to a heart attack or stroke. Normally, your body produces all the cholesterol you need, so it's a good idea to keep your daily cholesterol intake to below 300 milligrams.

Fat and Happy:
How Much Fat Can You Safely Eat?

In general, to be your healthiest, aim for having no
more than 30 percent of the calories in your total diet
as fat and 8 to 10 percent as saturated fat.

To figure out how much fat you can safely eat
every day, determine the number of calories you normally eat and follow the chart below:

Saturated Fat and Total Fat:
How Much Is Safe?

If you eat . . .	You can have . . .	including . . .
1,200 calories	40 grams of total fat	13 grams of saturated fat
1,500 calories	50 grams of total fat	17 grams of saturated fat
1,800 calories	60 grams of total fat	20 grams of saturated fat
2,000 calories	67 grams of total fat	22 grams of saturated fat
2,500 calories	83 grams of total fat	28 grams of saturated fat

If you're like most people, you've learned that
you'll need to rework your current way of eating to
trim some fat and cholesterol. On the pages that
follow, we give you 365 ways to do just that. We hope
you think of them as 365 ways to change your life—
and health—for the better.

Shop 'Til You Drop (the Fat)

1

Question: What's the difference between three pats of butter and the same amount of apple butter?
Answer: About 12 grams of fat and 33 milligrams of cholesterol. Fruit butters are fat free!

2

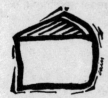

Cheese It on Cheese. One ounce of cheddar cheese has 9 grams of fat. Grab reduced-fat cheddar at 6 grams or try part-skim mozzarella instead at only 5 grams of fat.

3

Upper Crust, Lower Fat. A raisin bran muffin has 10 grams of fat and 30 milligrams of cholesterol; one slice of raisin bread has only 2 1/2 grams of fat and no cholesterol.

> No man is lonely while eating spaghetti; it requires so much attention.
>
> —*Christopher Morley*

4

Better Skip the Croissant. A 4-inch croissant may have as many as 4 teaspoons of butter, and a biscuit made from rolled dough can have as many as 9 grams of fat! Go for a plain bagel with only 1 to 2 grams of fat.

5

A Low-Fat Sandwich Is No Baloney. A typical baloney sandwich has 24 grams of fat. Switch to low-fat beef baloney or sliced chicken breast and trim the fat to just 3 grams.

6

Fishing for Fat. Buy tuna packed in water rather than oil. It'll save you 2 grams of fat on your next sandwich.

7

Let's Get Cereal. Most cereals are low in fat. The exceptions are cereals containing coconut, coconut oil, or nuts, so look for low-fat granolas!

8

Danish for Breakfast? Don't do it. It has more than 14 grams of fat and 26 milligrams of cholesterol. If you must, try the nonfat variety.

9

No Free Lunch. Steer clear of regular processed meats (luncheon meats) because 60 to 80 percent of their calories are from fat, most of which is saturated. Look for the low-fat variety with only 20 to 40 percent fat.

10

Hamburger Helper. Buy the deepest color of ground beef you can find. The darker the red, the less fat it contains.

11

Where's the Beef? It's not in the cuts marked "prime" or "choice." Choose "select" cuts of round steak, flank, sirloin tip, and tenderloin to trim the fat.

12

Round Ground. The leanest cuts of beef are round (eye of round, top round, bottom round, round tip), loin (top loin), sirloin, and extra-lean ground beef.

13

Miss Piggy's Finest. Lean cuts of pork are tenderloin, center loin roasts, and loin chops. Be sure to trim the fat on the edges.

14

It's Revealing. Almost any cut of veal is lean if it's trimmed of fat, except for the breast, ground veal, and veal cutlets.

15

Lamb Chopper. The leanest lamb cuts are leg, loin roasts and chops, and foreshank. Remember to trim the fat before cooking.

16

Organ Stop. Limit yourself to eating organ meats, such as liver, only occasionally. They're rich in iron and low in fat but abundant in cholesterol.

17

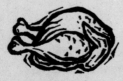

Everybody Loves a Skinny Chicken. Choose the leaner light meat (breast) rather than the fattier dark meat (legs and thighs). And always remove the skin before cooking.

18

Hot Tip for Frozen Entrees. Many of the calories come from fat, so choose entrees containing 10 grams or less of fat per serving.

19

The Whole Story. Look for the term "whole-grain" on ingredients labels. That means the grain product still has all its natural nutrients, including a high fiber content.

20

Carbo Loading. You'll eat less fat if you fill up on carbohydrates. Make grains, potatoes, whole-grain breads, rice, pasta, vegetables, and legumes almost 50 percent of your diet.

21

There's More Than One Way to Skin a Chicken. Remove the skin from poultry before cooking or grinding. Ask the butcher to clean the grinder to remove any fat left over from previous grindings. If you're roasting a chicken, it's okay to leave the skin on during roasting, then remove it before eating.

22

Liquid Assets. Buy margarine that lists liquid vegetable oil as the first ingredient. It should contain no more than 2 grams of saturated fat per tablespoon.

23

Soup It Up! Can the regular cream-based soups and chowders. Try the low-fat versions. Or choose

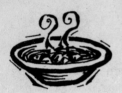

soups based on broth or vegetables instead, such as minestrone, vegetable, split pea, lentil, potato-leek, Manhattan clam chowder, and clear onion soup.

24

Here Comes the Sun. If you'll be using sun-dried tomatoes, buy the dry ones, not the ones packed in oil.

25

Hooked on Cheese Sauce? Then cut the fat in half by mixing 1 package of frozen vegetables with cheese sauce and a second package without the sauce. Or use frozen vegetables with low-fat sauces.

26

Bread Winners! Invest in these low-fat breads and crackers: whole-wheat bread, corn tortillas, English

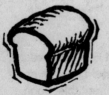

muffins, French bread, Italian bread, low-fat flour tortillas, low-fat whole-grain crackers, bagels, pita bread, pumpernickel bread, rye bread, and sourdough bread.

27

Bring Home the Bacon. If you absolutely must have bacon, try the leaner Canadian bacon or lean ham instead of regular bacon.

28

Soy Joy. Turkey bacon and bacon made from soy products have about half the total fat and a lot less saturated fat than pork bacon. Watch out for the amount of sodium, though. Many of these bacons are high in salt.

29

Love Mexican Food? Then look for fat-free refried beans in your grocery store.

30

Cocoa: Chocolate That Works Out. Did you know that cocoa powder is chocolate with most of the fat removed? When you crave chocolate, reach for recipes that call for unsweetened cocoa powder.

31

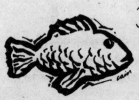

Fish Is a Good Catch. It's generally low in fat, especially saturated fat. Try to eat fish a few times a week.

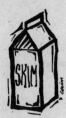

32

The Straight Skinny on Milk. Take a look at the fat content of different types of milk:

One Cup (8 oz.)	Total Fat (g)	Saturated Fat (g)	Cholesterol (mg)	Calories
Whole milk	8.2	5.1	33	150
2% reduced-fat milk	4.7	2.9	18	121
1% low-fat (or light) milk	2.6	1.6	10	102
Skim (or nonfat or fat-free) milk	0.4	0.3	4	86

33

The Butcher Knows Best. Some cuts of pork are truly lean; others are packed with fat. Check with your butcher for the leanest cuts.

34

Hot Dog Day. If you can't stay away from this all-American favorite, at least buy the ones labeled "fat free" or "low-fat." Regular hot dogs have almost 16 grams of fat each!

35

Lean and Mean. "Lean" on a meat package label lets you know that each serving of the product has less than 10 grams of fat, 4 grams of saturated fat, and 95 milligrams of cholesterol. Be sure to read the label for serving size.

36

Extra! Extra! "Extra Lean" on a label means that each serving contains less than 5 grams of fat, 2 grams of saturated fat, and 95 milligrams of cholesterol.

37

Exciting Salads. Salads don't have to be ho-hum. Add taste and texture with fennel, kohlrabi, daikon

radish, jicama, cilantro, arugula, radicchio, baby corn, portobello mushrooms, and Anaheim, banana, and sweet yellow bell peppers.

38

Guilt-Free Goodies. Nonfat chocolate syrup satisfies those chocolate cravings without the fat. Ditch the hot fudge and use this instead for cooking or toppings.

39

Fresh Is Best. Buy the finest and freshest ingredients so that your food will taste delicious and natural—without adding fat.

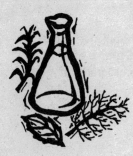

40

Last of the Big Spenders? If you're feeling flush, indulge yourself in gourmet flavor enhancers, such as raspberry and tarragon vinegars, capers, and fresh herbs.

41

Are You a Coco-Nut? When a recipe calls for high-saturated-fat coconut, buy coconut extract instead. It adds the flavor but none of the fat. You can also find reduced-fat coconut milk with about three-fourths of the fat removed.

42

Stock Portfolio. Always stock your kitchen with these classic flavor enhancers: garlic, ginger, mustard, onion, flavored vinegars, citrus juices and zests, and exciting herbs, such as fennel and cilantro.

43

Worth Its Salt. To enhance the flavor of low-fat foods, use freshly ground peppercorns and salt, ground from crystals in your own table mill. The taste difference will be astounding—and you'll use less salt than you will with an ordinary salt shaker.

44

Not the Same Old Grind. Get a nutmeg grinder and put it on the table. Use it in addition to—or instead of—salt and pepper. It makes fat-free food sing!

45

Believe in Basil. It adds flavor to tomatoes, potatoes, cucumbers, and squash.

46

Get Carried Away With Caraway. Caraway seeds will give new life to beets, cabbage, potatoes, and rye bread.

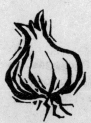

47

Garlic Won't Keep Vampires Away. But it's great for spicing up string beans, mushrooms, beans, tomatoes, and greens.

48

Take a Holiday From Hollandaise. Instead of high-fat sauces or dressings, squeeze lemon juice over asparagus, broccoli, spinach, and salads.

49

Savor Savory. Savory is a little-used spice that perks up beans, peas, lentils, salads, and vegetable juices.

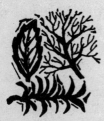

50

The Eyes Have It. Make your low-fat dishes look scrumptious with creative garnishes and edible flowers.

51

Tubby Tomatoes. Some bottled and canned tomato sauces have more than 7 grams of fat in a ½-cup serving. Look for a sauce with 3 grams or less of fat instead.

52

Put Your Big Temptations in Little Packages. If a premium ice cream splurge is irresistible, buy only a small dish or a cone. That way, you won't have any left over to tempt you the next day.

53

Don't Get All Wrapped Up in Fat. Filet mignon is a lean beef cut, but many supermarkets wrap it in bacon. Do your heart a favor by taking off the bacon before cooking.

54

Go Flavor Crazy! Feel free to run amok with almond, banana, lemon, rum, and peppermint extracts! They add a ton of flavor and not a trace of fat.

55

Fat Chance. Buy reduced-fat and fat-free versions of salad dressings. If you haven't tried them since they first came on the market, you're in for a pleasant surprise.

56

Chip Off the Old Block. Instead of buying potato chips, make bagel chips. Cut any flavor of bagel into 1/4-inch rounds (refrigerated or day-old bagels work best). Spread the slices on an ungreased baking sheet. Bake at 350°F for 10 to 12 minutes or until crisp and light brown.

57

"Cholesterol-Free." On a nutrition label, that means the product contains less than 2 milligrams of cholesterol and 2 grams or less of saturated fat per serving.

58

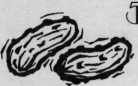

Get Pickled. Olives are high in fat. Choose pickles instead.

59

"Fat-Free." On a nutrition label, this is your clue that the product contains less than 1/2 gram of fat per serving.

60

"Reduced-Fat." If you see this on a product's package label, then the food item has 25 percent less fat than the regular version of the food.

61

Lite Up Your Life. When you see "Light" or "Lite" on a package label, it means the food has at least one-third fewer calories or 50 percent less fat per serving than the regular version.

62

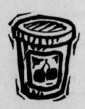

The Scoop on Yogurt. Custard-style yogurt contains 6 to 8 grams of fat per 1-cup serving compared with 0 to 4 grams in nonfat and low-fat yogurts.

63

Light on the Mayo. Regular mayonnaise contains 6 to 11 grams of fat per tablespoon. The light versions of these products contain 3 to 5 grams.

64

Sorry, Charlie. One-half cup of tuna salad made with oil-packed tuna and regular mayonnaise contains about 20 grams of fat. Instead, buy water-packed tuna and nonfat mayonnaise and save up to 18 grams of fat!

65

Cheers! Cream-based liqueurs contain up to 5 grams of fat per ounce. When choosing an after-dinner liqueur, decide on one that's not cream-based.

66

You Can't Pick It Up at the Grocery Store, But Attitude Is Everything. Even something as small as using 1 pat of margarine on toast instead of your usual 2 will save 4 grams of fat every time you do it. It's a small step, but every step counts. And all the steps together add up fast!

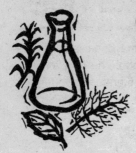

67

Herbal Infusion. Buy (or make) oil infused with herbs. It imparts a powerful flavor with just a few drops.

68

Last Line of Defense. If it isn't at home, you can't eat it. Avoid the temptation to buy high-fat items "just in case company drops in." Guess who'll end up eating it?

Sizing Up Servings

69

Double the Pleasure, Half the Fat. Eat half an oversized portion or split an entree. Large steaks, fajitas, pasta, and Chinese food can easily feed two people.

70

Nuts—In a Nutshell

Nut (1 oz.)	Calories	Fat (g)
Almonds, dry roasted	167	15
Cashews, dry roasted	163	13
Corn nuts	124	4
Macadamia nuts	199	21
Peanuts, dry roasted	164	14
Pecans, raw	190	19
Pistachios, dried	164	14
Sunflower seeds	162	14

> At a dinner party, one should eat wisely, but not too well,
> and talk well, but not too wisely.
>
> —*W. Somerset Maugham*

71

Cut Your Servings Down to Size. For healthy eating all you need is 3 ounces of cooked meat or poultry at a single serving. That's a piece of meat about the size of a deck of cards or half a chicken breast or a leg and a thigh.

72

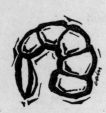

Shrimp Got a Bad Rap. Even though shrimp and crayfish have a tad more cholesterol than other fish, they're still low in total and saturated fat.

73

Daily Bread. Most adults need at least 6 servings daily of breads, cereals, and starchy vegetables, but what *is* a serving? Here are some serving examples: 1 slice of bread, 1 cup cooked rice or pasta,

1 cup flaked cereal, 1/4 cup nugget- or bud-type
cereal, 1/2 cup cooked cereal, or 1/4 to 1/2 cup starchy
vegetables.

74

Reality Check. You may think a bagel is 1 serving.
Think again. Today's jumbo bagels could be 2 to 3
servings.

75

The Yolk's on You. Eat no more than 3 or 4 egg
yolks per week. Count most baked goods as 1/2 an
egg yolk per serving.

76

Watch Out! A restaurant-size portion of pasta could
be 3 to 6 servings. Pay close attention to the amount
you're eating. Take leftovers home for lunch the
next day.

77

Bowl Yourself Over. Depending on the size of your
bowl of cereal, it could be 2 to 4 servings.

78

What's One Serving? One medium piece of fruit,
1/2 to 1 cup cooked or raw vegetables, or 1/2 cup fruit
or vegetable juice is one serving.

79

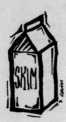

Dairy Diary. One serving of dairy products is 1 cup skim or 1% milk, 1 cup nonfat or low-fat yogurt, or 1 ounce nonfat or low-fat cheese.

80

Nice to Meat You. One serving is 4 ounces raw meat, poultry, or fish (3 ounces cooked).

81

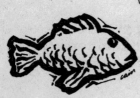

Big Fish, Small Serving. Here's an easy way to figure the serving size of fish: It's the same size as a 3-ounce can of tuna.

82

Munchie Mania. Watch how much you're eating at snack time. It's easy to sit down to watch the movie of the week and polish off an entire bag of potato chips. Instead, remove the number of chips you plan to eat from the bag, seal up the rest, and put them back in the pantry.

83

How Many Grams of Total Fat Should You Eat in a Day?

If you eat . . .	You can have . . .
1,200 calories	40 grams of fat
1,500 calories	50 grams of fat
1,800 calories	60 grams of fat
2,000 calories	67 grams of fat
2,500 calories	83 grams of fat

84

Keep Your Intake of Saturated Fat at 8 to 10 Percent of Total Calories. So, if you normally eat 1,500 calories a day, you can have 13 to 17 grams of saturated fat.

85

A New Angle on Meat. Slice meat on an angle and fan it out on the plate to make a small portion look twice as large.

86

Crackers Count. One serving is not the whole box. Read the label and munch accordingly.

Cooking for a Healthy Heart

87

Put Your Popcorn on a Diet.
Instead of making regular popcorn
at 4 grams of fat per cup, air pop it
at less than 1 gram of fat per cup.
For extra flavor, lightly spray the
popcorn with vegetable oil spray
and sprinkle garlic powder on it.

88

Olé, Amigos! Make your own tortilla chips *without
fat.* Cut corn tortillas into six wedges each. Spread
wedges on an ungreased baking sheet and bake at
400°F for 10 to 11 minutes. Then chow down with
spicy salsa.

89

Self-Basting Turkeys Are for the Birds. Save the
fat and baste with low-fat chicken broth instead.

> **Kissing don't last; cookery do!**
>
> —*George Meredith*

90

A Little Light Reading. Inspect ingredients labels carefully for fat and avoid high-saturated-fat oils such as coconut, palm, and palm kernel oil.

91

Wanted: Help-Your-Heart Vegetable Oils. Choose safflower, corn, sesame, sunflower, soybean, olive, or canola oil.

92

Cocoa-Loco. Make your next cup of cocoa with skim milk. You'll ditch 95 percent of the fat.

93

Taco Tricks. Cut the fat in ground beef before adding your taco seasoning. After browning, put the beef in a colander and run hot water over it for several minutes. Guess what goes down the drain!

94

Chestnuts to You. In your stir-fried cashew chicken recipe, use low-fat, low-calorie water chestnuts instead of cashews. Doing so cuts 13 grams of fat and 163 calories per ounce!

95

Vive la French Toast! Instead of using eggs to make French toast, use bananas and soy milk. Take 1 cup of chopped ripe bananas, 1 cup of low-fat soy milk, 2 or 3 tablespoons of all-purpose flour, and add vanilla, cinnamon, and nutmeg to taste. Blend bananas and milk in a blender until very smooth. Add other ingredients and blend. Dip bread and grill in a nonstick pan until golden.

96

Chicken With a Kick. Give your roast chicken zing by basting it with a mixture of powdered mustard and chicken broth.

97

Making Brownies? Read the box for suggestions on lower fat options.

98

How Now Skim Cow. When the recipe calls for
1 cup of whole milk, use 1 cup of skim milk instead.

99

The Big Chill. Stewing cooks some of the fat out of
meat. Cook it a day ahead and put it in the refrigerator to chill. This will make the fat rise to the top. Then
you can remove it before reheating.

100

Fear of Frying. Instead of high-fat frying, try steaming, baking, broiling, stewing, poaching, roasting, or
microwaving.

101

Celebrity Roast. Instead of
sautéing vegetables, oven-roast
them whole. This brings out their
natural sugars and gives them a
delicious flavor. Try onions, carrots,
asparagus, or an unpeeled head
of garlic.

102

Picnic Fare. Steam 10 new potatoes, chop 3 stalks of celery, and
toss with 2 tablespoons of mustard
and a small jar of capers. Yum!

103

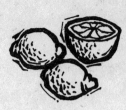

Give Your Salad Dressing a Workout. Make your own reduced-fat salad dressing by using apple, orange, grapefruit, lemon, or tomato juice in place of half the oil.

104

Buttermilk Blessings. If you're into creamy salad dressings, make your own using low-fat buttermilk as the base. It has only a quarter of the fat of whole milk!

105

Cream Team. Combine low-fat buttermilk with a low-fat soft cheese for a seriously creamy dressing.

106

Salad Style. If dairy is not your style, tofu is an exciting nondairy option for making salad dressings creamy.

107

Yogurt Spread. Place a double layer of paper coffee filters inside a strainer. Set the strainer over a bowl. Place nonfat yogurt that doesn't contain gelatin in the coffee filters. Refrigerate for 8 hours or overnight. Makes a smooth, thick spread you can use in place of cream cheese or sour cream in many recipes. You

can also save the whey that drains out of the yogurt
to use for baking in place of skim milk.

108

It Takes Two to Mango. Try mango chutney as a
topping for grains.

109

Hitting the Sauce. Need a sauce for rice? Try
1/4 cup of cooked beans blended with 1 cup of water
or tomato juice.

110

Hot Off the Grill. Grilling allows the fat to drip away
from meat as it cooks!

111

The Thrill of the Grill. If you usually fry your vegetables or cover them in cheese sauce, grill them
instead. Start with zucchini, portobello mushrooms,
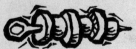 and cherry tomatoes.
Cooked outdoors, they're
delicious—and have no fat!

112

Veg Out. Instead of regular cheese for omelets, use
blanched vegetables, such as chopped broccoli or
spinach.

113

Microwave! It's easy, fast, and requires no added fat.

114

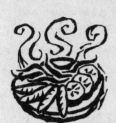

Veggie Magic. Lose the fat but keep the flavor by steaming vegetables only until they're tender-crisp. Add herbs, spices, or broth for extra allure.

115

Cookies and Cream Milkshakes. In a blender combine 1 pint vanilla, chocolate, or coffee nonfat or low-fat yogurt and 1/4 cup skim milk. Cover and blend until smooth. Add 2 chocolate sandwich cookies. Cover and blend just until cookies are coarsely chopped. Makes two 1-cup servings.

116

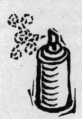

Spray Away. Use nonstick vegetable oil spray in place of oil or margarine for coating pans.

117

Splash It On. Try fruit-flavored or balsamic vinegar on steamed greens and other strong-tasting vegetables.

118

Heart-Smart Canapés. Add your favorite spices, fruit, or vegetables to light cream cheese, Neufchâtel cheese, or nonfat cream cheese for a low-fat spread for crackers or bagels.

119

In Love With a High-Fat Recipe? Experiment. Try paring down the amounts of butter, margarine, mayonnaise, and oil by a third or half. It rarely hurts the recipe but always helps your heart.

120

Casserole Clue. For casseroles with less fat, more fiber and nutrition, and a delicious taste, use wheat germ, bran, or whole-wheat bread crumbs in place of buttered crumbs as a topping.

121

Sly Spaghetti. Reduce the fat in your meat sauce for spaghetti by cutting the ground beef in half and adding sautéed mushrooms and zucchini. Even the kids won't notice!

122

Wok Right In. Stir-frying is the Asian version of sautéing. A wok is ideal because it cooks food in a small amount of oil—usually peanut oil because it won't smoke at high temperatures.

123

Let Fat Take the Heat. Broiling is brilliant. Why? Because cooking meat on a rack under direct heat allows fat to drip away. For extra flavor, marinate steaks, fish, or chicken before broiling.

124

Minimum Fat, Maximum Flavor. Roasting is a slow, dry-heat method of cooking that cooks the fat out of meat. Just season your meat and place it fat side up on a rack in an uncovered roasting pan. Baste with a fat-free liquid, such as wine, tomato juice, or lemon juice. Roast to desired doneness in a preheated 325°F oven.

125

Beef Up Your Low-Fat Cooking Repertoire. Braising is a slow-cooking method that tenderizes tough cuts of meat. To braise, just brown meat on all

sides using a little vegetable oil or vegetable oil spray.
Then season, add ¼ to ½ cup liquid, cover pan
tightly, and simmer.

126

Into the Frying Pan. But not to fry. To sauté. This
cooking method allows you to cook meat or vegetables over high heat with little or no fat. With sautéing, you cook the food in broth, wine, or a little
vegetable oil spray in an open skillet. You constantly
agitate it, causing it to jump (the French word *sauter*
means "to jump") to keep it from sticking. Sautéed
garlic, onions, peppers, and mushrooms add flavor to
many main dishes.

127

No Poaching. Except when you want a low-fat
meal. Then poaching in nonfat or low-fat liquid is a
great way to cook. Place a single layer of chicken
or fish in a shallow, wide pan and barely cover with
liquid. You can use water, water seasoned with
herbs and spices, skim or 1% milk, broth, or a
mixture of white wine and water. After cooking, you
can reduce the liquid and then thicken it to make
a sauce.

128

Salad Days. Cut down on fat in creamy salad dressing by mixing it with plain nonfat or low-fat yogurt or
skim milk.

129

Baking With Your Heart in Mind. For each egg in any baking recipe, substitute 1/4 cup applesauce or canned pumpkin or half of a mashed banana. You'll get the same amount of moisture without the fat.

130

Fruit for Fat. When your baking recipe calls for oil or shortening, substitute prune baby food instead. You'll get 75 percent of the moisture that oil or shortening furnishes without the fat. Try this with your favorite gingerbread recipe.

131

Baking With Corn. Pureed fresh corn will substitute handily for fat in baking recipes when the finished product needs extra texture. Sweet fresh corn adds fiber, moisture, and no fat—and that's the sweetest thing of all!

132

Jalapeño Hens. Preheat oven to 375°F. Take 2 (1- to 1 1/2-pound) Cornish game hens, split lengthwise and skinned, all visible fat removed. Rinse and pat dry. In a small saucepan, heat 1/2 cup jalapeño jelly over low heat until warm. Place hen halves cut side down in a single layer in a shallow roasting pan. Spoon about half the warm jelly over the hens. Roast, uncovered, for 30 minutes. Baste with jelly and cover loosely with foil. Continue roasting for 15 minutes or until hens are tender and no longer pink. To serve, spoon remaining warm jelly over roasted hens. Garnish with orange slices, if desired. Serves 4.

133

Crackdown on Crusts. Make your pies without crusts. (That's where most of the fat is!) Just choose a filling that's firm, such as pumpkin or refrigerated berries.

134

Nut So Wise to Eat That Pie. Pecan pie with whipped cream has 32 more fat grams than apple pie with low-fat frozen yogurt.

135

Tofu to the Rescue! Use soft tofu instead of cream cheese or eggs in cheesecake, custard, and mousse. Just be sure to double the spices and flavorings.

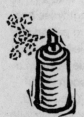

136

Better Butter. Try butter-flavored spray and granules to add butter flavor without the fat.

137

Tub Time. Use tub margarine rather than stick margarine or butter.

138

Look Sharp. For shredded cheddar cheese topping, use the sharp version. You can use less cheese and still get the cheddar flavor.

139

Egg Yourself On. Instead of a 3-egg omelet, try blending 1 whole egg and 2 or 3 egg whites. Or use egg substitute to equal 3 eggs.

140

Pasta Promise. You don't have to add oil to the water when cooking pasta. Just put the sauce on the pasta as soon as it's drained and it won't stick together.

141

Low-Fat Garlic Bread! Cut the head off an entire bulb of jumbo garlic and bake for 275°F for 25 minutes. Pop the cloves out and mash into a paste. Spread it on French bread and pop it in the toaster oven until brown. Voilà!

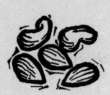

142

The Nuts and Bolts of Baking.
Reduce the amount of nuts in
cooking and baking. Better yet,
leave them out once in a while.

143

Love Hash Browns for Breakfast? Get the ones
made with no oil and brown them in a nonstick pan
with a little vegetable cooking spray until they're
crispy.

144

Share and Share Alike. Eat a mini-portion of
dessert or share a dessert with friends. Eat slowly.
Enjoy every bite!

145

Meatless Meals. Try baked eggplant sandwich
filling. Just preheat your oven to 350°F and slice an
eggplant about 1/2-inch thick. Spread 1 tablespoon
of low-fat pasta sauce on each slice and bake on a
vegetable-oil-sprayed baking sheet for about half
an hour.

146

A Hot Tip. Nonfat mayonnaise not your favorite?
Perk it up with a little hot sauce.

147

Measuring's a Must. Always measure oil in recipes, even if you like to "wing it" without measuring cups and spoons. It can save you a lot of fat without compromising quality or taste.

148

Get the Point? Skewer and grill green or red bell peppers, cherry tomatoes, zucchini, and onions to

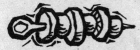 serve with lean steak rather than covering it with a butter sauce.

149

Bread Buster. Try hot yeast breads without any butter or margarine on top. Ummm . . . delicious.

150

Two New Buzzwords. Eat your bread with honey or maple syrup instead of butter or margarine.

151

Music to Your Mouth. Stir-fry a medley of frozen vegetables.

152

No-Fat Dessert. Core an apple, add a mixture of 1 tablespoon brown sugar and 1/8 teaspoon of cinnamon, and bake at 350°F or microwave on high until soft.

153

Chicken Little. A little skinless chicken or lean meat can go a long way in stir-fries, shish kebabs, stews, soups, and sauces. The flavor options are endless.

154

Fajita Faves. Making fajitas from poultry or lean skirt or flank steak? Save some of the meat to add to a main-dish tossed salad the next day.

155

Gelatin Surprise. Mix fruit and/or shredded carrots into flavored gelatin.

156

Zingy Cheese Snacks. For a rich-tasting snack, smear a dab of Dijon mustard on melba toast or whole-wheat crackers. Top with 1 ounce of part-skim mozzarella cheese.

157

Cottage Cheese With an Attitude. Try mixing pretzel pieces and nonfat or low-fat cottage cheese.

158

Sour Power. Whip low-fat cottage cheese to make a "sour cream" for potatoes or creamy salad dressings.

159

Dip Into Salsa. Veggie dips don't have to be high in fat. Try Mexican salsa for a different taste.

160

Spuds Are Buds. Potatoes aren't fattening. One medium-size baked potato with skin contains about 220 calories and is fat free. Go easy on the toppings, though. The fat grams in butter, margarine, sour cream, and cheese can add up fast! Nonfat sour cream or yogurt and butter-flavored sprinkles can add moisture and flavor without fat.

161

Potato Power. Don't thicken soups and sauces with a roux (a mixture of fat and flour). Use grated raw potato. It works as well but without the fat.

162

In the Thick of It. You can also thicken vegetable soups with barley.

163

Salsa Fiesta. Make your own delicious low-fat salsa by mixing diced fresh tomatoes with diced fresh onions, green peppers, cilantro, and chilies.

164

Give Greens the Green Light. Don't flavor greens with pork. Try a splash of flavored vinegar instead.

165

A Sassier Salsa. Mix chopped fresh or canned fruits (such as apricots, peaches, pineapples, or mangoes) with chopped tomatoes, chopped red onion, and minced garlic for an accompaniment to chicken or fish.

166

A Quick Thicken. Pureed starches thicken just about anything. Add pureed cooked dried beans, pasta, or mashed potatoes to soups, sauces, and gravies. They thicken with no fat.

167

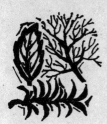

Cut and Dried. Dried herbs are concentrated, so use less of them than fresh herbs. In general, 1/4 to 1/2 teaspoon of dried herbs equals 1 teaspoon of fresh.

168

Undercover Fruit. Use moist ingredients to make up for oil. For example, add pineapple to stir-fries and bean dishes or add plumped raisins (made by soaking them in water for a few hours) to curry dishes.

169

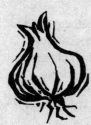

Garlic, the Spice of Life. Sauté 2 cloves of minced garlic in 1 teaspoon of olive oil. Stir into hot vegetables.

170

Don't Stick Around. Nonstick cookware lets you cook without much oil. Try it!

171

Get Steamed. Get a stainless-steel or bamboo steaming rack for nonfat cooking.

172

Heard It Through the Grapevine. Toss a handful or two of raisins into your rice during the last 5 minutes of cooking. The fruit will add a sweet zing and extra fiber.

173

A Grate Blend. To save fat, mix equal parts of low-fat or nonfat cheese and regular cheese. The combination will melt, and it will add much less fat and cholesterol than you'd get from using regular cheese by itself.

174

Quick and Easy Breakfast. For something hot and different in the morning, try cottage-cheese-and-cinnamon toast. Toast 1 slice whole-grain bread. Spread ¼ cup cottage cheese on top. Sprinkle with ¼ teaspoon cinnamon and ½ teaspoon sugar. Place in toaster oven or under broiler until topping bubbles.

175

Try a Little Tenderness. Marinating meat can help tenderize it and add flavor without adding fat. Here's an easy meat marinade: Mix 2 tablespoons light soy sauce, ¼ teaspoon hot pepper oil or ⅛ teaspoon cayenne pepper, 2 finely minced garlic cloves, ½ cup sherry, and 1 teaspoon grated fresh ginger. (If you're watching your salt, you can reduce or leave out the light soy sauce.)

176

Chef's Secret. Create a meat marinade from nonfat or low-fat salad dressings, flavored vinegars, wine, picante sauce or salsa, and citrus fruits, such as lemons, limes, and oranges.

177

Feeling Your Oats. Cut your fat intake by stretching your ground beef or turkey with starchy fillers, such as dry quick-cooking oatmeal, cooked rice, mashed potatoes, finely chopped or shredded vegetables, or bread crumbs.

178

Shorten the Shortening. Trim the fat by replacing part of the shortening in a recipe with applesauce or apple butter. It's super for cookie recipes.

179

Super Substitution. Use plain nonfat or low-fat yogurt instead of oil in brownie recipes.

180

Heart-Smart Tomato Sauce. Buy canned crushed tomatoes. Simmer with minced onion, plenty of garlic, black pepper, and classic Italian herbs, such as basil, oregano, and rosemary. Bravissimo!

181

Breakfast Booster. Cook hot cereals with extra water so they'll be creamier without adding milk or butter.

182

Cantaloupe Smoothie. Instead of a creamy, high-fat milkshake, puree cantaloupe in a blender. Delicious—and no fat!

183

Pasta Primo. Top your pasta with fresh vegetables simmered in low-sodium broth with herbs and spices. Put 1 tablespoon of Parmesan cheese per serving on top. This adds a ton of taste but only about 30 calories and less than 3 grams of fat.

184

Meal in a Minute. Turn a plain old salad into a one-dish meal by adding leftover chicken breast, lean roast beef, or reduced-fat ham; potatoes, pasta, or rice; and lots of veggies or some mandarin oranges, strawberries, or raspberries.

185

Can the Fat. Using canned chicken broth? No problem. Just refrigerate it first, then skim off the fat.

186

Groovy Gravy. Low-fat and delicious. Blend 1 tablespoon of cornstarch with 1 cup of defatted low-sodium broth in a jar with a tight-fitting lid by shaking until smooth. Heat remaining broth in a saucepan and add the blended liquid. Simmer until thickened.

187

Bravo! Instead of serving pasta with butter or pesto, top it with marinara sauce and a little Parmesan cheese.

188

The Pastabilities Are Endless. In fact, pasta doesn't need a sauce at all. Dress it up with chopped, julienned, and sliced vegetables of different textures and colors.

189

Soaked to the Skin. Use nonfat or low-fat Italian dressing as a marinade for meat, poultry, and vegetables.

190

Blender Magic. Pureed vegetables make fabulous sauces. Try eggplant with lemon or beans pureed with roasted garlic and hot peppers.

191

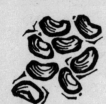

Bean There, Done That. Cook and puree beans or other legumes to make soups without cream or high-fat thickeners.

192

Turkey Surprise. Replace the ground beef in a recipe with ground turkey. There's no real taste difference as long as you increase the spices a bit to make up for the milder flavor of turkey.

193

Reggae Rice. Combine black beans and rice with chili powder for a Caribbean-style dish.

194

Kiss the Baker. For a low-fat cake frosting, blend skim-milk ricotta or low-fat cottage cheese and thin it with juice, honey, rum, or extracts.

195

Sweet Nothings. Use powdered sugar as a frosting on cakes rather than cream frosting.

196

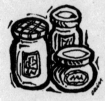

Beating the Breakfast Blahs. Puree nonfat or low-fat cottage cheese with chives, fresh fruit, or fruit preserves and spread on toast, bagels, waffles, or pancakes.

197

Pancake or Waffle Topping. Take 1 cup of fruit juice or water and thicken with 2 tablespoons cornstarch over medium heat, stirring so it won't get lumpy. Add 1 quart pitted cherries, 1/3 cup honey, a pinch of salt, and a dash of lemon juice. Heat until warmed through.

198

Cashing in Your Chips. Substitute raisins and chopped dried fruit for chocolate chips in baking.

199

Oriental Egg Substitute. Instead of eggs, try scrambling tofu. The cholesterol count is zero compared with 220 milligrams for each egg.

200

Hold the Mayo. Instead, add ketchup, mustard, horse-radish, chutney, salsa, or pickle relish to your sandwich to make lean meat, poultry, and fish sparkle. (If you're watching your sodium intake, note that some of these foods may be higher in salt than mayonnaise.)

201

Cheesed Off. Experiment with strong-flavored cheeses, like blue, Roquefort, Gorgonzola, and Gruyère. A small amount will add tons of flavor but not much fat.

202

Miracle Muffins. Make your own low-fat muffins using skim milk, egg whites, or egg substitute and substituting mashed bananas for oil.

203

Mixing It Up. If you're making packaged muffins from a mix, replace the added oil or shortening with fruit puree.

204

Super Soup. Instead of ham hocks, add roasted red peppers or smoked turkey to homemade pea or bean soups or stews for smoky flavor without the fat.

205

French Fry Fanatic? Then save yourself the fat and bake them. For oven french fries, scrub 4 large potatoes and cut into long strips about 1/2-inch wide. Place in ice water, cover, and chill 1 to 2 hours. Remove potato strips from water and dry thoroughly. Place strips and 2 tablespoons peanut or safflower oil in deep bowl and toss until potatoes are lightly coated with oil. Preheat oven to 475°F. Spread potatoes in a single layer in a shallow baking pan. Bake 30 to 35 minutes, stirring occasionally to brown on all sides. Serves 8.

206

Guest Dazzler. To make low-fat chocolate fondue, stir together 3/4 cup sugar, 1/2 cup unsweetened cocoa powder, and 4 teaspoons cornstarch in a small saucepan. Add 2/3 cup evaporated skim milk and cook over medium heat until thick and bubbly. Continue cooking for 2 minutes, stirring constantly. Don't cook too fast or at too high a temperature or the sauce can become lumpy. Dip fresh strawberries, bananas, pineapple chunks, or grapes into the warm chocolate. Only 4 grams of fat in the entire recipe!

207

Crunchy French Toast. It's low-fat, high-fiber, and delicious. Dip whole-grain bread in a mixture of egg substitute and wheat germ. Cook on each side till brown in a skillet coated with nonstick cooking spray. Dust lightly with powdered sugar.

208

Low-Fat Egg Salad? Yes! Combine chopped, cooked egg whites, light mayonnaise, chopped celery and red bell pepper, a dash of dry mustard, and freshly ground black pepper.

209

Ready to Roll. Freeze cooked brown rice and whole-wheat pasta in family-size portions. In the morning, remove a package and place it in the refrigerator to thaw. For a quick dinner, serve rice with a stir-fry or pasta with an Italian-style sauce.

210

Flying Colors. Combine green, yellow, and red vegetables for an eye-appealing plate. For example, acorn squash and peas look more appetizing together than broccoli and spinach. Try these color combos:

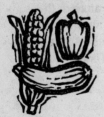 roasted red peppers and corn, sautéed zucchini and summer squash, grilled onions with red and green pepper strips, or kebabs of cherry tomatoes, pearl onions, and zucchini chunks, grilled or broiled.

211

Easy Does It. The long, slow, moist-heat cooking of slow cookers makes leaner, tougher cuts of meat juicy, tender, and flavorful.

212

Picnic Perfect. Make a coleslaw with healthy dressing. Mix 1/3 cup plain nonfat yogurt, 1 tablespoon apple cider vinegar, and 2 tablespoons honey. Toss with shredded cabbage and eat hearty!

213

Solving the Pie Crust Problem. Make a graham cracker pie crust with half oil and half fruit juice in place of melted butter or margarine.

214

The Pies Have It. Another great idea for low-fat pie crust is to combine 1/4 cup thawed apple juice concentrate with 1 cup nugget-type cereal. You can either blend it, crush it, or leave it whole. Press the cereal and juice mixture into a 9-inch pie pan, fill, and bake.

215

Why Whipped Cream? Often, chefs put whipped cream on desserts simply to counteract the sweetness. You can eliminate the need for whipped cream by making your pie, cake, or other dessert with less sweetener. Try reducing the sweetener by one-fourth.

216

Flour Power. Always use white cake flour or whole-wheat pastry flour when baking anything other than yeast breads. Cooks use fat in baking to break down gluten, and these flours have less gluten, so you can bake them successfully with no butter or oil—and they're still delicious.

217

The Proof Is in There. Make rice or tapioca pudding with egg whites or egg substitute and evaporated skim milk.

218

Monster Mash. For fluffy, no-fat mashed potatoes, simply mash steamed potatoes with a fork or hand masher, adding a little vegetable broth. Finish whipping with an electric beater, then add sweet Hungarian paprika, freshly ground pepper, and a dash of salt.

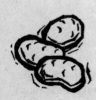

219

Food for Thought. Cook and mash Yellow Finn potatoes. They look buttered, but they're fat free!

220

Crust Creation. Here's an idea for a low-fat crust for a tofu quiche or vegetable pie. Cook short-grain brown rice by putting it in cold water and bringing it to a boil, then lower the heat, and stir occasionally. Press the sticky rice into a pie plate and fill it.

221

Fat-Free Breakfast Spreads. Take 8 ounces of softened nonfat cream cheese and add the zest (the colored part of the peel) of 1 orange or 1 lemon and 2 tablespoons of the juice.

222

Fat-Free Appetizer Spread. Take 8 ounces of softened nonfat cream cheese and add 1 clove of minced garlic, 1 teaspoon of dried basil or thyme leaves, and pepper. Or make a honey mustard spread by adding 1 packet of honey mustard salad dressing mix.

223

Banana-Kiwi Breakfast Shake. Combine in a blender: 1 medium banana, peeled and quartered;

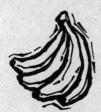

1 medium kiwi fruit, peeled and halved; 1 cup low-fat buttermilk; 6 ounces nonfat or low-fat fruit-flavored yogurt; and 1 to 2 tablespoons sugar (optional). Blend until smooth and serve. Makes two 1-cup servings.

Eating to Your Heart's Content

224

Do You Scream for Ice Cream? Yodel for nonfat frozen yogurt instead. (Saves 22 grams of fat and 240 milligrams of cholesterol per cup!)

225

Big Offender. One of the biggest sources of fat in the typical diet is salad dressing. (Two tablespoons has 19 grams of fat and 15 milligrams of cholesterol!) Try low-fat or nonfat salad dressings or lemon juice instead.

226

Breakfast on the Run. Try a little dry oatmeal and almonds with nonfat yogurt. Yum!

> Cooking is like love. It should be entered into with abandon or not at all.
>
> —*Harriet Van Horne*

227

Breakfast Parfait. Put nugget- or bud-type cereal in the bottom of a bowl, spoon on your favorite nonfat yogurt, and top with berries.

228

Pita Party. Eat a meatless lunch of pita bread stuffed with vegetarian chili, hummus, lettuce, and tomato or low-fat cottage cheese mixed with chopped apple and raisins.

229

Souped-Up Soup. For a thick no-fat soup, add cooked and pureed potatoes or rice!

230

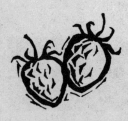

Milkshake Madness. Instead of an ice cream shake, make a fruit smoothie. Blend frozen bananas, strawberries, and a splash of fruit juice for a luscious shake with zero fat.

231

Fiber Fights Fat. Whole grains, fruits, and vegetables help lower cholesterol. Try brown rice instead of white rice and pumpernickel instead of white bread.

232

Just Desserts. Help your heart with low-fat desserts like angel food cake with sweetened sliced berries, pudding made with skim milk, nonfat cookies, warm fruit compote, poached pears with raspberry sauce, or baked apples with cinnamon.

233

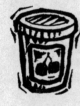

Snack Attack. When you simply must have a snack, go the low-fat route. Try frozen fruit bars, nonfat frozen yogurt, Italian ices, sherbet, sorbet, fresh or dried fruit, hard candy, or jelly beans.

234

Tater Topping. Crumbled bacon has almost 35 grams of fat per ounce. Try imitation bacon bits with only 4 grams of fat per ounce.

235

Lite Lunch. A regular-size hamburger has 11 grams of fat. A 3-ounce piece of grilled chicken has 3 grams of fat. Any questions?

236

Coffee Catch. Instead of cream or whole milk in your coffee, use evaporated skim milk. Same creamy taste—without the fat.

237

Breakfast of Champions? Fast-food egg sandwich at 8 grams of fat and 235 milligrams of cholesterol or a bagel with fat-free cream cheese at 3 grams of fat and 0 milligrams of cholesterol? You decide.

238

The Skinny on Fat. Fat is the most concentrated source of calories. It contains 9 calories per gram. Protein and carbohydrates contain only 4 calories per gram.

239

Salad Smarts. Salad bars can be full of hidden fat.
 Stay away from cheeses, marinated salads, pasta salads, and fruit salads with whipped cream. Choose fresh greens, raw vegetables, fresh fruits, garbanzo beans, and nonfat or low-fat dressing.

240

Cajun Cooking. If you like hot and spicy food, go ahead and be generous with the hot sauce. Your taste buds will be so busy, they won't know you've cut the fat.

241

What the Best-Dressed Potatoes Are Wearing. Low-fat salad dressing, mustard (Dijon, honey, or horseradish style), light soy sauce, nonfat or low-fat cottage cheese, steak sauce, starchy beans, salsa, or broccoli with reduced-fat cheese melted with skim milk.

242

Take a Stab at It. Dip the tip of your fork into salad dressing, then stab some salad. You'll have the salad dressing flavor with every bite, but your salad won't be drenched in it.

243

Tastes Eggsactly Like an Egg. Egg substitutes are made from egg whites, a little bit of vegetable oil, and some flavorings. They look and taste like whole eggs but are much easier on your heart. Try 'em!

244

Dressing for Success.

1 Tablespoon of	Calories	Fat (g)
Fat-free dressing	5–25	0
Lemon juice	0	0
Picante sauce	4	0
Balsamic vinegar	6	0
Fruit vinegars	6	0
Nonfat mayonnaise	12	0
Reduced-calorie, all types	15–40	2–4
Reduced-fat mayonnaise	50	5

245

Butter Blues. Look at the big difference between butter, margarines, and butter flavorings.

	Calories	Fat (g)	Saturated Fat (g)	Cholesterol (mg)
Butter (1 tbsp.)	100	11	7	30
Stick margarine (1 tbsp.)	90	10	2	0
Light tub margarine (1 tbsp.)	40	4.5	0	0
Butter-flavored spray (5 sprays)	0	0	0	0

246

Five Alive. Eat at least 5 or more servings of fruits and vegetables a day. Not only does they give you the vitamins, minerals, and fiber you need, they fill you up. No room for fat!

247

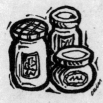

Make All-Fruit Spreads Your Bread and Butter. Instead of butter or margarine on toast, use all-fruit spreads, fruit butters, and even sliced bananas and strawberries.

248

Expecting Meat-Hungry Guests for Dinner? Serve them shish kebab. It's easy and elegant. You'll

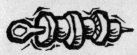

dazzle them with your culinary creativity while keeping meat portions to a minimum.

249

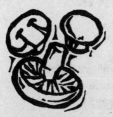

Meat Substitutes. Put eggplant, mushrooms, and sun-dried tomatoes in stir-fries, soups, sandwiches, or Italian dishes. They have the satisfying feel of meat without fat or protein.

250

It Isn't Just for Breakfast Anymore. Try a low-fat hot cereal at lunch or dinner for a change. Sweeten it with raisins or peaches canned in fruit juice.

251

Power Lunch. Trade that lunch-time sandwich for a baked potato or a baked sweet potato. Just keep the toppings low in fat.

252

Go With the Grain. Cook raw grains by themselves. Barley, bulgur, couscous, farina, grits (polenta), millet, and oat bran are vitamin packed and delicious.

253

Tutti Fruity. Top your cereal with fresh, frozen, canned, or dried fruit.

254

Banana Waffles? You bet. Pour any pureed fruit over pancakes and waffles for a taste treat.

255

Divided You Conquer. When you fill your plate, pile half with fruits and vegetables, use one-fourth for a starch such as potato or pasta, and fill the last one-fourth with 3 ounces of lean meat, poultry, or seafood.

256

Moveable Feast. Carry a single-serving can of fruit packed in fruit juices for a delicious no-fat snack.

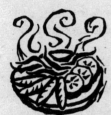

257

Veggie Dinner. Double or triple up on your vegetables and serve them with low-fat toppings.

258

Berry Good! For dessert, try a bowl of fresh berries topped with nonfat or low-fat yogurt.

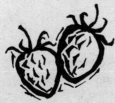

259

Food for the Angels. For a luscious low-fat "shortcake," mix strawberries, blueberries, and blackberries with nonfat vanilla or strawberry yogurt and serve over angel food cake.

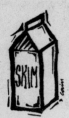

260

Got Milk? If you have access to a refrigerator at work, take a quart of skim milk to keep there. Enjoy a glass of nutrient-packed skim milk rather than a fast-food milkshake.

261

Powder Power. Keep nonfat dry milk in your cupboard. When reconstituted double strength and served cold, it's delicious.

262

Meatless in Seattle. Skip the meat in a meal or two this week. Make sure your meatless meals are well balanced by including whole grains, beans or peas, lots of vegetables and fruits, and nonfat or low-fat dairy products.

263

Veggies on Ice. Frozen vegetables that have been partially thawed make interesting snacks. Try corn, peas, or any others. Kids love the crunch!

264

Once Served, Twice Shy. Serve your plate at the kitchen counter and leave the serving bowls (or pots) there. That way you'll be less tempted to go back for seconds.

265

Bagel Benefits. Use nonfat or low-fat cream cheese instead of regular cream cheese on bagels.

266

Better Biscuits. Try low-fat biscuit and baking mixes. You may not be able to tell the difference!

267

Get Wise on Fries. A 2½-ounce serving of french fries has nearly three times the calories and nearly twelve times the fat of a 2½-ounce baked potato.

268

Check Out These Stats on Chips.

Potato Chip	Calories	Fat (g)
Regular chips	150	10
Reduced-fat chips	140	6.7
Baked chips	110	1.5
Fat-free chips	110	less than 1

269

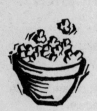

Popcorn Potential. Regular microwave popcorn has 3 to 7 grams of fat in a 2-cup serving. Light microwave popcorn has 1 to 2 grams of fat in 2 cups.

270

Tasty Pops. Season your air-popped popcorn with herbs or sprinkle on Parmesan cheese.

271

What's the Big Squawk About Fast-Food Chicken? A fried chicken breast and drumstick has a whopping 23.8 grams of fat. The same amount of rotisserie chicken (baked or broiled without skin) has 7.1 grams.

272

Diversionary Tactics. If you tend to snack on high-fat foods, have some low-fat snacks on hand for when you get the munchies.

273

Peanut Power. Hooked on peanut butter? Try mixing it with a filler, such as cooked carrots. You'll still get the taste but use so much less.

274

Go Greek. Try reduced-fat feta cheese. It crumbles nicely over soups and salads. And the flavor is luscious!

275

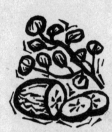

Also Good for High Tea. Just because it's a sandwich, you don't have to use meat. Try a watercress or cucumber sandwich instead.

276

A Fungus Among Us. Grilled portobello mushrooms remind many people of steak and are terrific served on a bun!

277

Sometimes You Feel Like a Nut. Chestnuts are delicious and, unlike other nuts, fat free!

278

Nuts About Nuts? Then get the taste but lose the fat. Try toasting cooked chickpeas topped with your favorite seasoning.

279

Ice Cream Quest. In the never-ending search for fat-free desserts, try a banana-sicle. Insert a sucker stick into a small peeled banana and freeze overnight. It tastes like banana ice cream but has no fat!

280

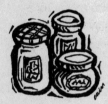

Super Snack. Make a dip for fruit with 8 ounces of plain low-fat yogurt, 3 tablespoons strawberry fruit spread, and 1/2 teaspoon cinnamon.

281

Got a Craving? Instead of a 1 1/2-ounce chocolate bar, try a 1 1/2-ounce chocolate-covered peppermint patty. You'll save 9 grams of fat and about 100 calories.

282

Chocolate to the Rescue! Out of the blue, you get a chocolate craving. Don't panic. Instead of reaching for a full-size candy bar, pick up only three bite-size pieces of chocolate candy. That'll quell your urge to splurge.

283

Chocoholic? Two tablespoons of chocolate syrup contain about 73 calories and less than $1/2$ gram of fat. Most hot fudge sauces, however, contain 10 grams of fat per $1/4$ cup. Of course, you *can* buy fat-free chocolate syrup or use just a tiny bit of the real thing!

284

Low Fat, High Fiber. Add kidney beans or chickpeas to a lettuce or spinach salad.

285

Yum! Try whole-wheat macaroni and chickpea stew in tomato sauce.

286

Pasta Pleaser. Cut down on calories, fat, and cholesterol in baked pasta by using vegetables instead of meat. Try zucchini lasagna, spinach-stuffed rigatoni, or broccoli and low-fat cheese-stuffed shells.

287

Pretzel Power. Hard and soft pretzels are great low-fat snacks.

288

Start Your Blenders. Pour in a little fruit juice, add bananas, strawberries, and a little pineapple. Voilà! A no-fat fruit smoothie. If you like it a little creamier and more like a shake, start with skim milk.

289

Do Your Crunches. Always keep plenty of fresh fruits and vegetables on hand. Raw veggies with nonfat or low-fat dip and fruit with low-fat cottage cheese make healthy snacks.

290

The Smooth Solution. Always make pudding with skim or 1% milk.

291

In the Red. Eating fish with as much cocktail sauce as you want instead of 2 tablespoons of tartar sauce saves up to 8 grams of fat.

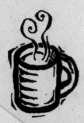

292

Winter Warm-Up. If you drink a cup of hot apple cider instead of a cup of cocoa, you'll save more than 3 grams of fat.

293

Flavor Brigade. Rice cakes have no fat and are great snacks. You can try a different flavor every day for a week and still not run out of flavors!

294

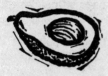

It's Not Easy Being Green. Trim the fat in guacamole by stretching the avocado with pureed broccoli or nonfat sour cream.

295

Nonfried Frijoles. For healthier Mexican food, cook and spice chili beans. Then whip them in a blender or food processor. You get the fluffiness without the fat.

296

Flavor Saver. For a light, sweet flavor, cook vegetables in fruit juice. For example, turnips and carrots are great cooked in orange juice.

297

Sticks to the Roof of Your Mouth. If you're a peanut butter freak, cut the fat by mixing in cooked, pureed garbanzo beans. They'll carry the flavor and texture but add zero fat.

298

Southwestern Spread. Blend chickpeas with lime juice, oregano, cilantro, and chipotle chilies.

299

Ham It Up. To add the flavor of ham to bean and pea soups, but not the fat, season with sage or meatless bacon-flavored bits.

300

Free What? Fat-free, but not calorie-free, candy includes licorice, most hard candies, gummy candies, and jelly beans.

301

Nonfat Ice Cream Sandwich. We knew that would get your attention! Sandwich a thick slice of nonfat frozen yogurt between 2 chocolate-flavored rice cakes. It's a cold, crunchy, and creamy treat that's easy on the heart.

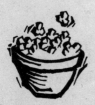

302

Sweet Snack. Drizzle honey or molasses over plain, air-popped popcorn. It's like caramel corn you can eat with a spoon.

303

Belly Up to the Bar. Eat a fruit juice bar instead of an ice cream bar and save up to 25 grams of fat.

304

Entertaining? Instead of bowls of nuts, set out a trail mix of pretzels, dried fruits, cereals, and just a few chopped nuts.

305

Down With High-Fat Crackers. Rather than put your appetizers on high-fat crackers, use mushroom caps or make croustades. How? By cutting the crusts off white bread, rolling the bread with a rolling pin until it's as thin as a pie crust, cutting the slices into rounds that will fit in the bottom of a muffin tin, and baking the rounds for 10 minutes at 250°F.

306

Barely There Spray. Put oil in a spray bottle and give your salad a squirt to help the seasonings stick to the greens. You'll get minimum oil but maximum flavor.

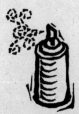

307

Chomp! Use a butter-flavored spray on corn on the cob. It tastes the same but saves about 10 grams of fat over buttered corn.

308

High Brow, Low Fat. Try steamed, fresh artichokes and dip the leaves into a sauce made of nonfat yogurt with either Dijon mustard and a dash of cayenne pepper or lemon juice and a dash of hot pepper sauce.

309

Be Grate-ful. Grate a small amount of Parmesan cheese over hot vegetables. Big flavor, little fat.

310

Breakfast Japanese Style. Try rice, miso soup, spicy nori (seaweed), or steamed or stir-fried vegetables with either fish or tofu—and tea. It's fabulous on cold mornings.

311

Pig Out? If you eat a lot of high-fat foods at one meal, all is not lost. Go fat-free at another meal or two to compensate.

The Inside Scoop on Dining Out

312

Fast-Food Fake-Out. Which has more fat, a plain hamburger or a fried fish sandwich? Surprise! The fish sandwich, at 16 grams. A plain regular hamburger has 11 grams. A plain kid's burger has only 9!

313

Life in the Fast-Food Lane. It's not so dangerous if you know how to drive. Example: Choose grilled chicken (about 3 grams of fat per serving) or chicken salad (5 grams of fat per serving) instead of fried chicken nuggets (3 grams of fat per piece).

314

Even If You Don't Own a Rover. Ask for a doggy bag when you order a large meal and set aside a take-home portion before you dig in.

> *The discovery of a new dish does more for human happiness than the discovery of a new star.*
>
> —*Anthelme Brillat-Savarin*

315

On Your Side. Ask that sauces and dressings be served "on the side."

316

To Dine For. Choose restaurants that have heart-healthy options. You'll find them flagged right on the menu. If you don't see what you want, ask the waiter to have your dish prepared as fat-free as possible.

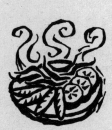

317

The Spa Who Loved Me. Look for restaurants featuring "spa," "contemporary," or "California" cuisine; generally their food is lower in fat.

318

Advance Planning. Decide what you're going to have before you get to the restaurant. That way, you'll be less tempted by fat-filled menu choices.

319

Jump to It. Be the first to order, if possible. This helps prevent temptation.

320

Leave Off the Fat. Ask the waiter to leave the chips, french fries, or other high-fat side dishes off your plate. If possible, get fruit or a vegetable instead.

321

Beware the Breadbasket. Watch out for pre-buttered bread and rolls with a glaze. These fats add up. Ask for plain bread and rolls instead.

322

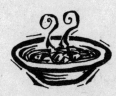

Fill 'Er Up. Begin your meal with water and salad, raw vegetables, or clear soup. If you know they won't be available, start with a snack like this before you leave for the restaurant.

323

Menu Mojo. Look for these tip-offs to low-fat menu items: "au jus" (in its own juices), "baked," "broiled" (with lemon juice or wine), "fresh," "grilled," "poached," "lean," "roasted," and "steamed."

324

Make a U-Turn. Run, don't walk, away from foods described as "au gratin" (in cheese sauce), "buttered," "breaded," "casserole," "creamed," "fried," "crispy," "hash," "rich," "sautéed," or "scalloped." They all mean "high fat."

325

Pizza Plan. Order double vegetables instead of double cheese on your pizza.

326

Fast-Food Breakfast. Instead of the artery-clogging breakfasts served at most fast-food restaurants, choose orange juice and an English muffin (2 grams of fat). In a pinch, try pancakes with syrup and no butter or margarine (4 grams of fat).

327

No Greater Tater. Ask for a small or medium baked potato rather than a potato the size of Idaho.

328

Oh, Waiter! If the restaurant gives you a bowl of chips, fried noodles, or nuts, ask the waiter to take them away. Or put a few on your plate and have the rest removed.

329

Stick 'Em Up. A slice of bread or a couple of breadsticks (no butter) are good low-fat appetizers. But be sure to leave some room for your meal!

330

Size Up the Competition. Check portion sizes by measuring your food at home. That way, you'll know on sight if the portions served at a restaurant should be trimmed down a bit by leaving some on the plate.

331

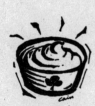

Be Assertive. Ask the waiter for what you want. Ask for margarine instead of butter, vegetables without butter, and plain toast.

332

Be Curious. Ask how food is prepared. Many restaurants are willing to cook to your specifications. If the fish is fried, ask if the chef can broil or bake it instead.

333

Vegetable Pleasures. Order a plateful of steamed vegetables instead of a meat-filled entree. You'll leave the table feeling full but not stuffed.

334

Sweet Endings. Order a fresh fruit plate with a low-fat muffin to end your meal and enjoy just a forkful of your dinner companion's rich dessert.

335

Hot Potato. A luscious, low-fat potato topping is 3 tablespoons of nonfat yogurt and 1 tablespoon of pimento cheese.

336

Muesli Mix. If you choose a higher-fat cereal such as granola, try mixing it with cereals lower in fat.

337

Read Closely. Create your own meal from the appetizer and salad side of the menu. Order your entree from the appetizer section to get a smaller portion or put two or three appetizers together to make a lunch or dinner. You can sample several foods but have less food overall.

338

Pizza Party? Before you dive in, grab a few paper napkins and blot up the oil that's sitting on the melted cheese. This will save you several grams of fat per slice.

339

Decisions, Decisions. Special occasion dinners often include a cocktail, an appetizer, and a dessert. Decide ahead of time to choose just one of the three.

340

Orange You Glad? You can save fat by choosing a fruit sorbet.

341

Be Reckless. Leave some food on your plate. The Clean Plate Club has fallen out of favor.

342

Hold the Bacon. Cut the fat on sandwiches by omitting the bacon, mayonnaise, cheese, and special sauces. Instead, use mustard, tomatoes, lettuce, pickles, and onions.

343

Small Changes, Big Difference.

	Typical order	Modified order
Sandwich	Specialty burger	Regular hamburger
Side order	Large french fries	1/2 small order french fries
Beverage	12-oz. soft drink	Unsweetened iced tea
Dessert	Milkshake	Low-fat frozen yogurt
Total fat	64 grams	15.5 grams
Saturated fat	25.2 grams	16.1 grams
Cholesterol	150 milligrams	44.5 milligrams
Calories	1,436	475

344

Cater Your Own Restaurant Meal. Order a
vegetable side dish, rice side dish, dinner roll, a
vegetable-based soup, and fruit with frozen yogurt
for dessert.

345

Sweet as Pie. One-eighth of a pecan pie contains
24 grams of fat, 1/8 of a chocolate cream pie contains
about 17 grams of fat, and 1/8 of an apple pie
contains about 14 grams of fat.

346

Cut to the Crust. The fat is in the pie crust, so just order single-crust pies. For ⅛ of a pie, it'll save you 7 grams of fat.

347

Can We Talk? If you have a health condition that demands a low-fat diet, it's a good idea to write it down and have the waiter pass your note directly to the chef. That way you don't have to rely on the waiter to find a time when the chef can really listen to the request.

348

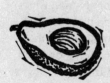

Smooth and Tempting. But go easy on the guacamole. Half an avocado has 15 grams of fat.

349

Go Below. Submarine sandwiches can be low in fat if you choose lean meats and lots of vegetables without oils and creamy sauces and spreads. And stick to the 6-inch size.

350

Chinese Takeout. Order wonton or hot and sour soup, steamed rice, and boiled, steamed, broiled, or lightly stir-fried dishes. Stay away from deep-fried dishes, fried rice, egg dishes, and salty sauces.

351

Maharaja Service. Indian food is generally low in fat and full of spices. Order the yogurt-based salads, tandoori chicken and fish, lentil or dal dishes, and pulka (unleavened wheat bread) or naan (without the butter). Watch out for foods cooked in coconut milk, cream, or ghee (clarified butter).

352

Asian Delights. If Asian food's your thing, keep it low in fat by ordering dishes lightly stir-fried with fresh vegetables and small amounts of meat, shrimp, or steamed fish. Try grilled or stir-fried wine-marinated meat dishes. Go for salads that combine shredded cabbage, chicken, pork, or shrimp with traditional spices (cumin, turmeric, or coriander) and peppers. Stay away from fried appetizers and entrees, creamy soups, and desserts made with coconut milk.

353

Greeks Bearing Gifts. Low-fat Greek dishes include plaki, fish that's cooked with tomatoes, onions, and garlic. Shish kebab is also good, along with

tzatziki, an appetizer made with yogurt and cucumbers. Order pita bread and those famous Greek salads, but ask the cook to leave the feta cheese, anchovies, olives, and dressing on the side.

354

Sacré Bleu! French cooking can be high in fat—
unless you know the ropes. Order items prepared in
the Provençale cooking style of southern France,

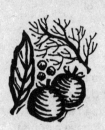

with tomatoes, onions, mushrooms, garlic, olive oil, and herbs.
These dishes usually feature fish
and vegetables. Choose delec-
table sauces made with wine,
such as bordelaise, but stay away
from the cream sauces, such as
béchamel.

355

Al Dente. When eating Italian, start with pasta. It's
naturally low in fat, so stay away from cream sauces
and pesto. Instead, ladle on tomato-based marinara
sauce, white or red clam sauce, or marsala wine
sauce. Or try pasta primavera. Watch out for fatty
meat- or cheese-filled pasta. End your meal with an
Italian ice.

356

Have a Yen for Japanese Food? Great, because
it's naturally low in fat. Try the nabemono, which are
Japanese casseroles; chicken teriyaki, which is
broiled in a sauce; and menrui, the noodles often
used in soups. Dishes with tofu are extremely nutritious and low in fat. Steer clear of deep-fried dishes
like tempura and high-sodium soups and sauces.

357

Shake, Rattle, and Roll. Milkshakes are swell, but they have as many as 14 grams of fat. Ask for low-fat shakes made with nonfat frozen yogurt and skim milk. They have as little as 1 gram of fat.

358

Put the Freeze on Fat. Fruit-filled snack pies contain as much as 15 grams of fat. For dessert, have a nonfat vanilla frozen yogurt cone instead and save yourself more than 14 grams of fat, or have a nonfat frozen yogurt sundae and save more than 12 grams of fat.

359

Ragin' Cajun. For the hot and spicy side of life, try these low-fat Cajun favorites: red beans and rice, Cajun rice, yams, greens, and cornbread without butter. Low-fat entrees include jambalaya or gumbo, blackened or baked fish, and boiled seafood dishes. Walk away from dirty rice, bisques, étouffées, and dishes made with andouille or boudin (sausages), a roux, or anything deep fried.

360

Jolly Mon. Caribbean dishes are low in fat as long as you stay away from coconut and cream-based soups, bisques, or fried dishes. Instead, try jerked meats; broiled, grilled, steamed, or boiled seafood; red beans and rice; rice with pork or shrimp; stuffed fish; and dishes with a fruit-based sauce. Traditional jerked meats are sun-dried in long strips and are salty. So if you're watching your sodium intake, go easy on this type of meat.

361

For Better or Wurst. To most people, Eastern European means beef goulash, chicken fricassee, schnitzel, and sausages. Well, it doesn't have to. Try rice-stuffed cabbage or peppers, yogurt-based borscht or fruit soups, and knishes filled with vegetables. For a main dish, ask for poached fish or poultry.

362

South of the Border. Mexican food is everybody's favorite, but some of it packs a high-fat wallop. Stay away from nachos, tortilla chips, guacamole, taco salads in a fried shell, refried beans, flour tortillas, and avocado soup. Turn down the chimichangas, flautas, taquitos, tamales, quesadillas, cheese en-chiladas, chiles rellenos, and huevos rancheros. Instead, order black beans or black bean soup, cantaloupe soup, ceviche, corn tortillas, gazpacho, salsa, and tortilla soup. For main dishes, choose arroz con pollo, mesquite-grilled chicken, anything wrapped in a soft corn tortilla, or fajitas minus the flour tortillas.

363

Magic Carpet Ride. If you love Middle Eastern
food, order couscous, baba
ghanouj, hummus, dolma, lentil
soup, pita bread, rice pilaf, tab-
bouleh, fattoush, and kufta as a
main dish. Fly past falafel, kasseri,
kibbeh, and meat pies.

364

Buffaloed? Resist the temptation to order chicken
wings. They're mostly fat with very little meat.

365

Short Stack. At the salad, taco, or potato bar, use a
smaller plate so you can't stack as much food on it.
This can help limit the fat and calories that end up on
your plate.

There's someone at every party who eats all the celery.

—*Kin Hubbard*

Don't Shy Away From Commitment

Now that you know 365 ways to eat less fat, we hope you'll make these tips a lifelong habit. Why? Because it's your best bet for living free of the ravages of heart disease and stroke.

Of course, this will take commitment on your part. And sometimes it's easy to think you're committed when you really aren't. It's like the story of the chicken and the pig. They were in the barnyard discussing what it means to be committed.

The chicken said proudly, "I give eggs every single morning—I'm committed."

"Giving eggs isn't commitment, it's participation," countered the pig. "Giving *ham* is commitment."

At the American Heart Association, we wish you the kind of commitment that will give you a lifetime of health, happiness, and delicious eating.

> **Where there's smoke, there's toast.**
>
> —*Old saying*

Index